EYE MELANOMA

A GUIDEBOOK FOR PATIENTS

RAJIV ANAND, MD, MS, FRCS

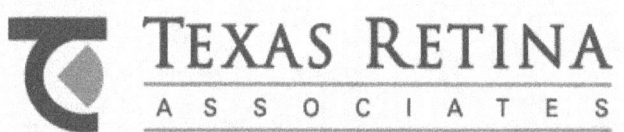

DALLAS, TEXAS

Copyright, Rajiv Anand MD
First Edition 2016

Dedicated to

Our patients

with eye melanomas

for their courage

and trust

EYE MELANOMA
Guidebook for patients and families
Contents

Foreword

Melanoma is a rare cancer of the eye that can cause loss of vision, and sometimes loss of life. This serious condition often hides for months to years in the confines of the eye and quietly causes visual distortion, symptoms of flashing lights, and sometimes pain. The goal in management is early detection of the tumor and treatment to induce complete regression and to prevent systemic metastasis.

Over the years, there has been great success with recognition of melanoma at an early point, leading to timely treatment. Small malignant melanoma can closely resemble the more common, benign choroidal nevus or freckle that can sometimes transform into malignant melanoma. Research has lead to identification of clinical risk factors that help predict which nevus/freckle is likely to evolve into melanoma. More recently, there have been genetic mutations discovered in some melanomas that predict tumor activity and cause the doctor to monitor the patient more closely.

In this handbook, Dr. Anand has succinctly summarized current knowledge of eye melanoma for the patient. The chapters accurately describe for the patient the signs and symptoms of melanoma, office-based testing to confirm the tumor, and overview of various treatments. A discussion regarding treatment decisions, pros and cons, practical matters regarding vision, and what to anticipate in the future all fit into the spectrum of patient concerns. The scientific and emotional aspects of ocular melanoma are well described.

Perhaps one of the most sensitive parts of this handbook is the final chapter, written by a patient who happens to be an eye doctor. This patient developed melanoma and describes his fears, experiences, and personal achievement to beat melanoma from his perspective.

Fortunately most patients with melanoma of the eye do well, with long, healthy life. And fortunately, research is leading to improved care with better quality of life and vision for the patient. We congratulate Dr. Anand for his creative and touching handbook for patients with eye melanoma – a treasury of informational facts, thoughts, and positive thinking.

Carol L. Shields, M.D.
Jerry A. Shields, M.D.
Ocular Oncology Service
Wills Eye Hospital
Thomas Jefferson University
Philadelphia, PA USA

EYE MELANOMA

A Guidebook for Patients and Families

INTRODUCTION

It is devastating for any patient or a member of their family to be told that they have a cancer within their body. It is even scarier when the cancer is diagnosed in the eye.
The word "tumor" or "cancer" invokes the thought of dying and even worse, surviving but losing vision and going blind.

Over the years, my associates and I have seen and managed many patients with melanoma of the eye. This handbook is meant as a guide for the patient and their family through the trials and tribulations of the diagnosis and testing. Details of the options in the management of the tumor should provide some guidelines about the current research and treatment methods.

About 30-40 years ago the only treatment available and widely practiced was the removal of the eye that contained a tumor. This, of course, resulted in loss of the eye and all vision even though the eye had useful vision at the time of diagnosis. Also, this resulted in removal of some eyes that actually did not contain a malignant cancer, but instead had other conditions that mimicked a melanoma. With the advent of newer diagnostic techniques and better treatments, physicians came to realize that treatment could be conducted so the eye can retain useful vision and also not have surgery that removed the eye altogether.

There is a lot of information on eye melanoma when you do a "Google search". Unfortunately, some of the information is dated, or biased or just plain inaccurate. As with any life threatening or blinding disease, false claims of cures, alternative methods of treatment and 'natural therapy' can be perplexing to those that need guidance.
We hope that this handbook will provide help, support and a sense of purpose to make informed decisions about the course of the disease.
 This handbook is dedicated to all the patients with eye melanomas who have been affected and survived the disease and contributed to our knowledge about its management.

HOW DO I KNOW THAT I HAVE A TUMOR OF THE EYE?

Unlike other cancers in the body, tumors of the eye seldom produce sudden changes in function or cause pain. In general, melanomas are slow growing tumors and are discovered during a routine eye exam. There may be a prior history of a freckle (called choroidal nevus, see section on 'nevus') that was noted years earlier and now has changed into a growing lesion, i.e., a tumor.

Sometimes a patient may report loss of field of vision (example a blind spot), floaters or just plain blurred vision. It is a rare case when the eye will become bloodshot and painful, though this can happen if the patient has ignored the symptoms for a long time.

At times, a persistent redness may be noted by the patient in the corner of the eye, or a cataract may develop in that eye due to the presence of the melanoma.

Often the patient gets seen for a change in their glasses and during their exam a solid growth is noticed inside the eye, prompting a referral to a retinal specialist.

Eye MDs always encourage patients to have at least an annual dilated eye exam with their optometrist or ophthalmologist.

HOW IS A MELANOMA DIAGNOSED?

Your eye doctor will normally conduct a full eye exam including a check of your vision and will check the pressure of the eye to rule out glaucoma. They will then dilate the pupil with eye drops to get a look inside the eye. Utilizing a microscope or specialized diagnostic camera, the eye doctor can look into the back of the eye and note whether the eye condition is normal or abnormal. Several specialized tests are done which are listed below.

Slit lamp exam

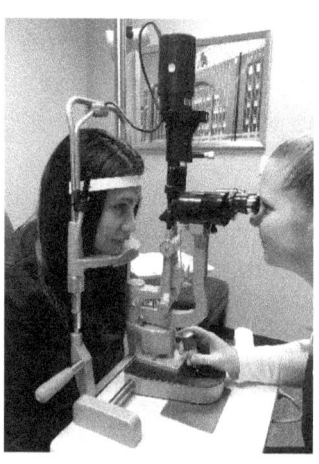

This is a standard, horizontally mounted microscope with a light that the eye doctor uses to examine both the front and back of each eye. This gives a magnified view of the eye with the light being used in different settings to examine the retina, the choroid and the optic nerve. *We emphasize that the pupil of the eye be dilated with eye drops so that a detailed exam can be conducted of the back of the eye. This is important so that nothing is missed.*

Binocular Indirect ophthalmoscope

This is a head-mounted instrument that allows the doctor to use a lens and allows a wide-angle view of the retina. Again, this is an important technique to examine all areas at the back of the eye.

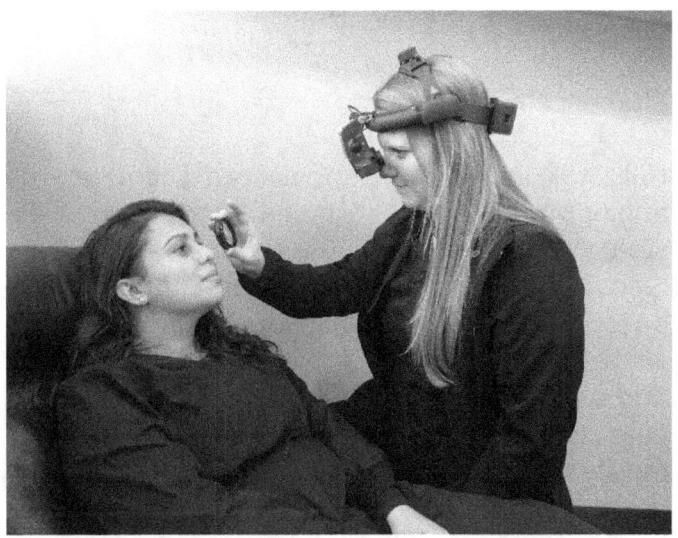

Photography

A specialized camera can be used to take a digital photograph of both the front and back of the eye. This gives a standardized view of the retina and the structures within the eye as well as provides a record for future comparison. These days, it is routine for optometrists to obtain wide-angle photographs of the back of the eye (Optomap images) and this provides a useful reference point for comparison in case any suspicious lesion is noted in the future. This also provides a benchmark to see if the lesion has changed over the course of the next few years.

Fluorescein Angiogram

Utilizing the same specialized camera, an angiogram can also be taken which reflects the status of the blood vessels inside the eye. Generally, a small amount (1 or 2 ml) of water-based, safe yellow dye (fluorescein solution) is injected into the vein in the arm of the patient, and as the dye circulates through the system, a blue camera light is used to obtain pictures of the back of the eye. As the dye circulates, the doctor can see the blood vessel pattern at the back of the eye and determine if there are abnormal blood vessels or differentiate them from hemorrhage or any other non-threatening lesion. Since a growing or active tumor requires a blood supply, these vessels will leak on the angiogram and provide more information on the components of the tumor.

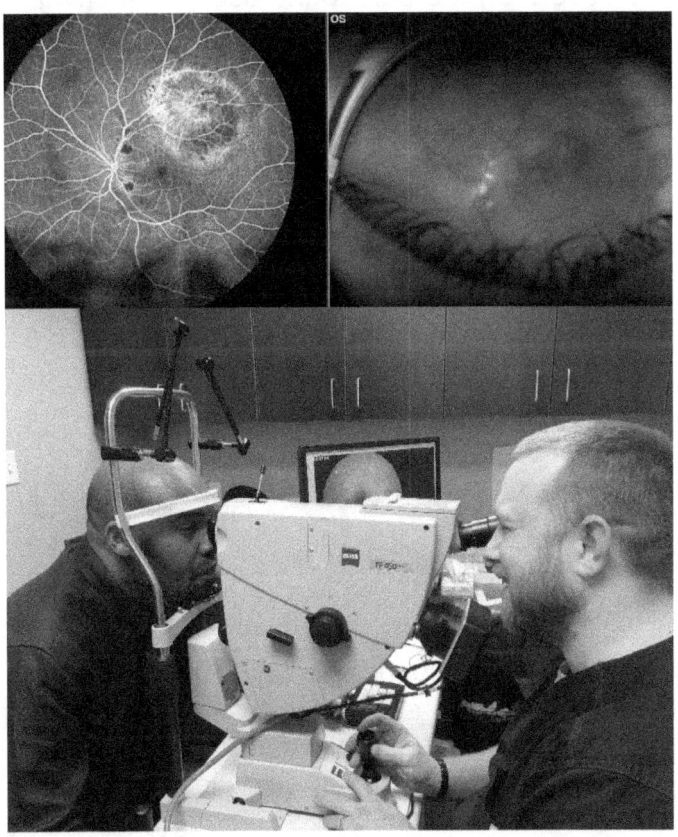

Ultrasound

A diagnostic ultrasound is a simple method of looking through the structures of the body, without the use of x-rays or chemical agents. Depending on how deep the ultrasound waves need to travel, different frequencies of ultrasounds are used and a specialized probe can be designed for the eye. This is a lot more sensitive than the ultrasound used for looking at pregnancies or within the infrastructures of the body (example: the abdomen).

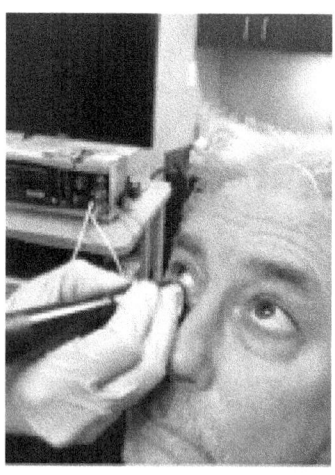

The ultrasound is located in a probe, which has a rapidly moving hand piece, and this is generally placed on the surface of the eye or through the closed eyelids to bounce a sound wave through the tissue structures. The sound waves that are reflected back by the structures inside the tissues give the eye doctor a pattern that allows him/her to differentiate between a growth or hemorrhage or a detachment of the retina. (B scan)

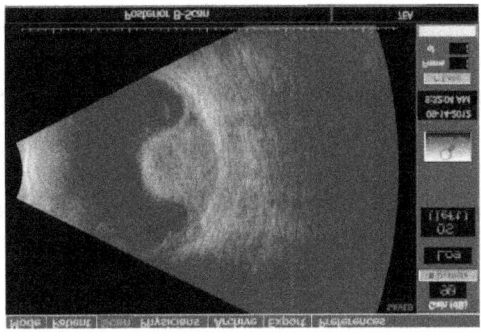

Similarly, an ultrasound that is accurately placed on the eye also reflects back waves that are used to measure the thickness of the lesion to within 0.1-0.2 mm. This is important when it comes time to determine which course of action to take for treatment and also to follow the progress or response to therapy.

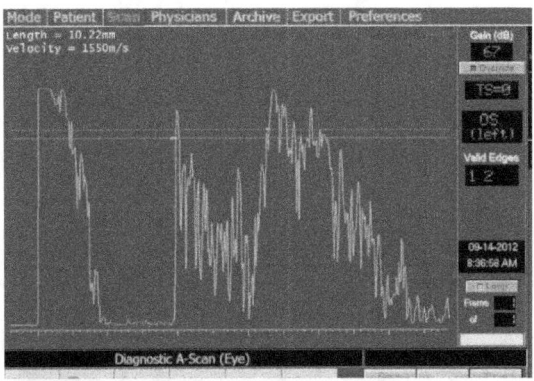

X-ray, CT (COmputerized tomography) scan, MRI (Magnetic resonance imaging) scan

Generally speaking, x-rays do not reveal a soft tissue growth in the body. Therefore, CT scan images are sometimes utilized to diagnose melanomas. Additionally, a CT scan is conducted to look at the liver and chest (see below). Magnetic resonance imaging (MRI) can also be used on some occasions if the doctor determines it is necessary, but this is not routinely employed to diagnose melanoma.

REVIEW : ANATOMY OF THE EYE

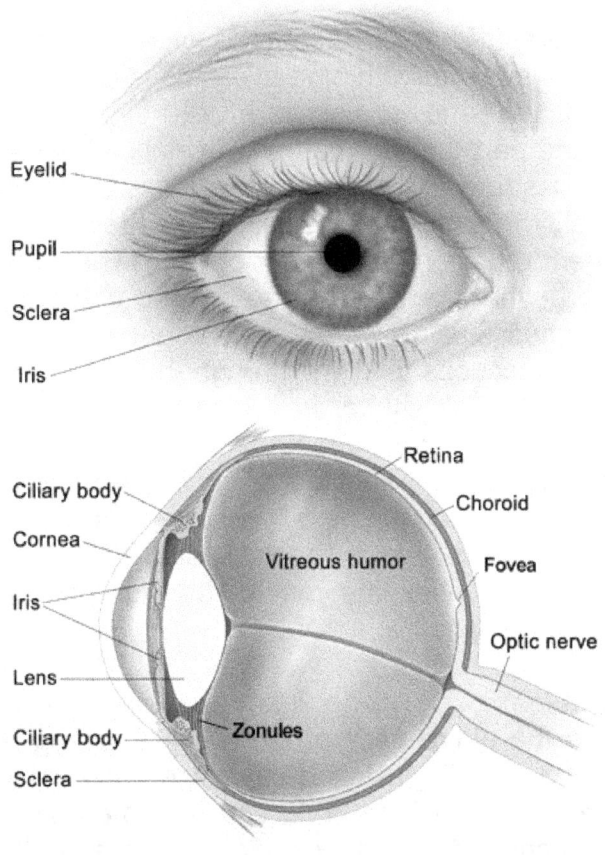

As shown in the diagram, the eyeball is held within the boney orbit surrounded by bones on all sides and protected by soft tissue that fills up the socket. There are six muscles that move the eye in different directions, up and down, side to side and rotation inwards and outwards. Most of the time both eyes work together like the front wheels of a car.

There are different layers on the eyeball. A clear transparent layer with blood vessels is called the conjunctiva and this covers the eye in the exposed part that is within the eyelids. A white, tough tissue called the sclera encloses the entire eyeball. The six muscles are attached in different positions on the sclera. The clear portion (what is visible as the colored portion) is the cornea that allows the light to enter the eye and also focuses the light through the pupil. The pupil is like the shutter in a camera that opens and closes depending on the amount of light that enters the eye. The diaphragm that makes up the pupil is called the iris and varies in color from blue to dark brown. The lens sits behind the pupil and focuses the rest of the light on the back of the eye.

The retina is the inside lining of the eye which covers the entire back of the eye like wallpaper covering up the inside of a soccer ball. The retina is a part of the brain and is formed by an out-pouching from the developing fetus in the womb.

Light focuses on the retina, visual signals are formed and the fibers of the retina go up the optic nerve to the brain where the image is processed. Any kind of swelling in the retina or fluid under the retina will cause a blind spot to appear causing a decrease in vision.

The choroid is the 'middle' layer that occupies the space between the retina and the outside sclera. This layer is rich in blood vessels and nourishes the retina as well as processing the vision. This is the layer where melanomas of the eye can occur. There are three distinct zones of the choroid. The first is the iris that forms the pupil. The second is the ciliary body, a muscle contracts and enlarges the pupil also suspends the lens behind the pupil. The third zone is the rear portion that encompasses the entire area of the retina called the choroid.

It is important to note that melanomas of the choroid in the front or the back of the eye have different implications as well as different means of management.

HELP! WHAT DO I DO NOW?
IMPORTANT QUESTIONS THAT MOST PEOPLE ASK AT THE TIME OF DIAGNOSIS

1. Will I lose my eye?
       Answer: Most of the time, the eye can be saved unless the tumor is very far advanced or too big to be treated. (See below)
2. Will it spread to the other eye?
       Answer: No.

3. Will it spread to the face and orbit?
    Answer: No. Melanomas do not spread outside the eye within the face or orbit (very rare, see below).
4. Will it spread to the brain?
    Answer: No.
5. Will I die?
    Answer: The workup after the initial diagnosis is important. Most of the studies have shown that melanomas tend to remain confined to the eye for quite some time. Majority of patients do well and continue to lead normal active lives. However, cancer of any kind anywhere in the body is unpredictable and continued care and surveillance over the rest of the patients' life is extremely important. This cannot be over emphasized!
    (See section below on gene expression and work up after diagnosis)

TREATMENT OPTIONS: WHAT TO DISCUSS WITH YOUR DOCTOR

After the initial shock of the diagnosis has worn off, it is always advisable to go back to the retina specialist for another visit and discuss the different treatment options that might be available.

The majority of the time the patients say "I don't want to lose the eye", and "I want to keep the best possible vision".

 Over the last few years the emphasis has been preservation of the eye and the maximum vision possible, and not to automatically consider removal of the eye.

Credit for this change in attitude of management goes to several researchers over the years and a large study conducted by the Nation Eye Institute called the Collaborative Ocular Melanoma Study (COMS). This study and its results are detailed in a section below.

The different treatment options available are listed below and will be discussed in further detail with the pros and cons of each under a separate subheading.

1. Enucleation
2. Plaque radiation therapy
3. Radiation – external beam therapy
4. Surgery to remove the tumor
5. Laser treatment
6. Observation alone and no treatment
(under extremely rare conditions)

ARE THERE SPECIALIZED CENTERS THAT TREAT EYE MELANOMAS?

There are specialized centers that deal with treatment of ocular melanomas. These centers specialize in the teaching hospitals of the country and your eye doctor should be able to advise you whether this is necessary and refer you accordingly. When making a decision to travel to these specialized centers, the patient has to keep in mind the cost of travel, the stay in a city outside their hometown, the cost of the coverage of treatment, and the strain on their families.

FIRST STEPS TO TAKE AFTER DIAGNOSIS
AND BEFORE MAKING A TREATMENT DECISION

A full physical exam with your general medical doctor is necessary. This includes chest and liver imaging either with a CT scan or MRI, blood tests that can be done to look specifically at the liver, and routine blood counts. As mentioned above, rarely is there imaging required of the orbits and brain, unless it is a very advanced or unusual case.

Why liver and lung?

The reason for looking at the liver and chest is that this is where preferentially melanomas of the eye tend to home outside the eye. Most patients know about melanomas of the skin, however, melanomas of the eye and skin have very little in common except for their name. Thus, melanomas of the skin tend to spread locally, whereas melanomas of the eye tend to go through the bloodstream to distant sites outside the eye, namely the liver and then the chest.

Since the eye has very rich blood supply, there are constant, little tumor cells that circulate in the bloodstream and they tend to home to the liver and chest. However, there is scientific evidence to show that the body sets up its own immune surveillance and mechanism that can keep these circulating tumor cells from invading or settling in any other organ, thereby providing some kind of defensive immunity.

More recent research utilizing gene expression studies show that Type 1a and 1b tumors are less aggressive in leaving the eye compared to Type 2 tumors.

However, if the tumor cells have already invaded the liver and lung, the treatment options become different and somewhat limited. Obviously, at that point both the liver and the eye have to be treated simultaneously (see below).

We always encourage the patient to form a long-term relationship with a cancer specialist who can then provide support and continued follow-up. Patients should be seen by their own doctor or an oncologist at six-month interval with exams and blood tests in the first few years. After that, they can be seen at longer intervals as deemed appropriate by the oncologist and also dependant on what the gene expression shows.

WHAT ABOUT A BIOPSY? HOW DO YOU KNOW THAT THIS IS INDEED A MELANOMA OF THE EYE?

This is an excellent question and many patients want to know how the diagnosis is established. Once again, this goes back to the research that has already been done as part of the COMS study and experience accumulated over the last 50 years. The COMS study showed that examination of the eye along with the tests listed above was capable of diagnosing the melanoma accurately 99% of the time. However, there are some instances where the tumor is so unusual that a biopsy to obtain a sample of the tissue may become necessary.
This is conducted by the retina specialist and in the operating room under anesthesia.

In the past, a large biopsy was risky because of the danger of causing bleeding or further loss of vision by putting a needle in the eye. However, newer techniques of surgery have allowed us to obtain a very small sample from within the tumor itself to conduct a microscopic analysis. A biopsy of this nature should only be conducted at a specialized center that does these all the time.

A biopsy of the tumor is also valuable in providing an indication of how aggressive the melanoma is. (Type 1 or Type 2 – see section on gene expression)

PRACTICAL ASPECTS OF DIFFERENT TREATMENT OPTIONS

1. Plaque radiotherapy
   Plaque radiotherapy is the most common form of treatment of eye melanomas and this treatment was tested in great detail by the COMS study. As part of the study, tumors were labeled small, medium or large. The results of the COMS were most helpful in the management of medium sized melanomas.

   The treatment consists of application of a radioactive source placed right on the surface of the white of the eye (sclera). This is a treatment that is conducted in the operating room since it requires accurately placing the radioactive source on to the surface of the eyeball. Most times the surgery can be done on an outpatient basis (day surgery).

The source of the radioactive material most commonly used in the United States is radioactive iodine (Iodine-125). In Europe, other radioactive sources such as ruthenium or palladium are used as the source of radiation. There is generally no difference in the efficacy of any of these radioactive materials.

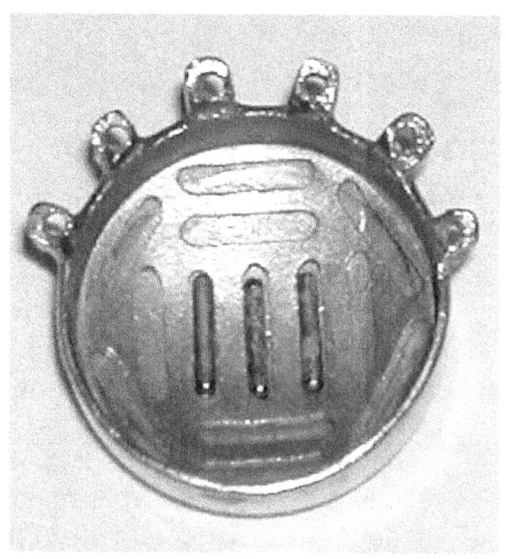

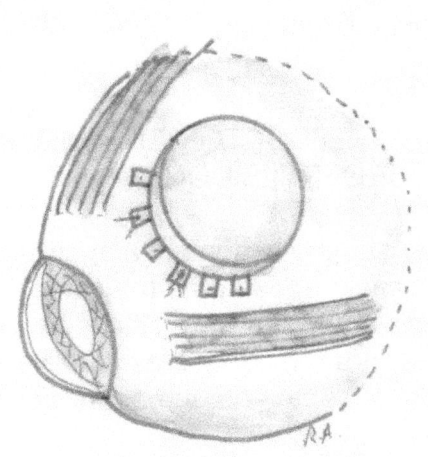

RADIOACTIVE PLAQUE STITCHED TO SCLERA

The radioactive plaque is made out of a shell of either gold or other rare material that can accommodate a plastic dummy into which the radioactive seeds are inserted. The plaque and the radioactive sources are individualized for each eye so that they deliver a very accurate dose of radiation to the eye tumor. This is calculated by the radiation physicist (depending on the radio-isotope used) using a mathematical formula as well as the strength of radioactive seeds and the thickness of the tumor.

Since the outside of the plaque has a thicker layer of metal, the radiation is directed inside the eye. This causes very little external damage so patients do not lose their eyelashes or eyebrows or have discoloration of the skin.

DISCUSS WITH THE DOCTOR THE DETAILS ABOUT HOW SURGERY IS DONE

Most of the time, surgery is done in a specialized center and the patient goes home the same day. The radioactive plaque can stay stitched to the surface of the eye from 3–7 days as it delivers a steady radiation dose to the tumor inside the eye.
Removal of the plaque is done in he operating room as well. While it takes an hour or more to stitch the plaque into the correct anatomical space over the surface of the eye, removal of the plaque can be done fairly efficiently and quickly. This may take only about 30–45 minutes.

During the time the radioactive plaque is stitched to the eye, the patient is advised to stay indoors and not be exposed to a dusty environment. We also recommend that because of the effects of radiation, the patient keep away from young children and anyone who might be pregnant. The radiation safety officer will give you very accurate and specific guidelines about the safety while the radiation plaque is on the eye.

During this process, it is expected that the eye will be red, inflamed and swollen (imagine a metal the size of a quarter stitched to the surface of the outside of the eye). Most times, cold packs placed on the skin outside and simple painkillers can keep the eye very comfortable during the 3-7 days the plaque is stitched to the eye. Once the plaque is removed, the swelling and redness on the outside of the eye will gradually decrease and most times the patients will use artificial tear drops, some antibiotic drops or ointment for a few weeks before they can be discontinued.

FOLLOWUP AFTER PLAQUE RADIOTHERAPY

Most times your doctor will re-examine the eye within the first couple of weeks to allow the eye time to heal. Thereafter, patients will need to be seen at 2-3 month intervals in the course of the first year. Ultrasound measurements and examination of the eye will be conducted as per the doctor's discretion, though we don't expect to see much shrinkage of the tumor till about three months following plaque removal.

So, do not expect the tumor to disappear in the first few weeks. In fact, studies have shown that the ideal response is a slow shrinkage of the tumor over 12-24 months to a stable, flattish scar.

Generally speaking, the patient needs to be seen at least 4 times a year in the first 2 years, after which if the tumor is regressing satisfactorily, the visits can be dropped down to every 6 months, and later once a year.

It is important that patients realize that this is a life-long observation and follow-up plan. The reason for the continued observation is that in case there is a chance that the tumor shows some degree of small growth, it can be treated with an additional radioactive plaque or supplemental laser therapy.

EXTERNAL BEAM RADIATION THERAPY

Proton beam radiation applied through an external source to the patient's eye achieves the same results as a plaque placed on the surface of the eye to treat the melanoma. There are a few specialized centers where this treatment can be done. The two major centers that have specialized in this treatment are in Boston and San Francisco.
The treatment consists of 2 or 3 external beams of radiation that are focused on the eye, and the patient undergoes multiple sessions of this treatment lasting several minutes at each session. Initially, careful measurements will be taken where the tumor is located in the eye and small markers will be placed on the surface of the eye to accurately pinpoint the angle at which the radiation beams enter the eye. Thereafter, the patient has a special mold made for his/her

head so that there is no movement of the head while the radiation is being applied.

Follow-up after external beam radiation is similar to treatment with radioactive plaque therapy and the results, as well as complications, are similar.

WHAT ARE THE SIDE EFFECTS OF RADIATION TREATMENT

As with any treatment that destroys tumor tissue, there are side effects to the surrounding healthy tissue. The most common is radiation retinopathy (see separate section), optic nerve damage if the tumor is located very close to the nerve at the back of the eye. Cataract does occur in eyes where the radiation is directed to the front part of the eye and this can be corrected with surgery and a lens implant. Retinal detachment may occur in some eyes but this too can be repaired with surgery. Unfortunately, a small percentage of eyes can develop high pressure and a painful glaucoma after a few years resulting in delayed loss of vision. In these cases, the eye may ultimately have to be removed.

SURGERY TO REMOVE THE TUMOR

Good question: why not just cut out the tumor, especially if the vision is good and the mass is confined to the eye?

So, surgery, while practically feasible has significant complications. (Imagine trying to remove only the yolk from a soft-boiled egg without losing any of the white AND preserving the egg shell!). Small tumors of the iris and ciliary body (front part of the eye), have been removed with some success but the complication rates are still much higher than radiation therapy. Surgery for larger tumors of the choroid has a very high rate of complications including retinal detachment and hemorrhage.

OBSERVATION : NO INTERVENTION

This is a rare option that we choose for a very small, select group of patients. Most of the time the patients are either very ill or have other complicating medical conditions, say bad heart disease or are very elderly. Since melanomas of the eye are slow growing and if the patient chooses to have no intervention because they cannot undergo even the lightest form of anesthesia, a choice of just observing and following the tumor can be considered.
 Most patients can and should be treated; it is very rare that this option is chosen and in general, not recommended.

FOLLOWUP AFTER TREATMENT: HOW OFTEN AND WHAT WILL BE REQUIRED OVER THE COURSE OF THE YEARS.

The patient needs to remember that from the moment of diagnosis to the treatment and throughout the follow-up, they should be guided carefully by their ophthalmologist as well as their oncologist. As noted above, the patient will be followed very closely over the course of the first year and if serial exams show that the tumor is shrinking down satisfactorily, the follow-up exams after the first few years will be less frequent. However, it is extremely important that you continue to be seen by your ophthalmologist at regular intervals even several years after the treatment has been successfully completed.

The reason for this is that there can be delayed reaction to the radiation, namely radiation retinopathy, damage to the optic nerve or cataract formation. Some of these conditions can be treated and therefore it is important that continued examination of the eye is conducted.

Once the initial exam and diagnosis has been made, the oncologist will most likely examine the patient once every 4-6 months during the first two years. This may consist of just blood tests or, alternatively, CT scans of the chest and liver once or twice a year. At times an ultrasound of the liver may be sufficient. After 2-3 years of follow-up, the oncologist may determine that just an annual exam is necessary.

We strongly suggest that the patient establish a long-term relationship with their primary doctor and oncologist for continued follow-up. This is regardless whether the eye is removed or the eye is treated with radiation.

WILL I NEED CHEMOTHERAPY?

Chemotherapy is generally not indicated in the treatment of melanoma of the eye. In the future, as more research trials are available, your oncologist may determine whether immune-boosting agents or any other drugs may become necessary during the follow-up period.

RADIATION RETINOPATHY

Radiation treatment is directed right over the eye and into the depth of the tumor to kill off the dividing cells. Once the active, dividing cells within the tumor have died, the surrounding cells in the eye will produce a reaction that will kill and absorb the remaining cancer cells. However, since the radiation treatment does not discriminate between healthy cells and tumor cells, there can be effects on the surrounding retina and adjacent optic nerve.

Most of the time, this results in gradual decrease in vision due to loss of blood circulation causing radiation retinopathy or swelling of the optic nerve. Cataracts can also develop but the cataracts can be treated very easily with surgery.

If the tumor is small and located further from the optic nerve and macula (center of the retina) then there may be no ill-effects from the radiation even several years after treatment.

Current trials are underway to reduce the side effects of radiation therapy. Your EyeMD should be able to determine whether injections of agents into the eye can be helpful in reducing the swelling or damage from radiation as you continue your follow-up in the future.

COLLABORATIVE OCULAR MELANOMA STUDY (COMS)

A brief summary

In the mid 1980's, eye melanomas were managed by different physicians in many different ways, some opting for immediate removal of the eye while others with radiation treatment. Long-term survival rates were reported to be good or bad and there was no consensus as to how best to treat different sizes of tumors.

By this time a lot of data were available from established experts in melanoma centers in Philadelphia, Boston, San Francisco and in the UK that showed that radiation treatment worked in many cases and was able to save useful vision. Controversy existed in the 'medium-sized' tumors: whether to treat or to remove the eye.

The National Eye Institute (NEI) sponsored a multi centered, randomized trial of newly diagnosed melanomas. Patients were followed closely for twenty plus years and after careful analysis of lots of different data, several scientific papers were published.

The tumors were divided into three categories: small, medium or large. Small tumors were observed till they grew, large tumors were promptly treated by removal of the eye. The emphasis of the study was on the 'in-between' or medium tumors where management was controversial.

After diagnosis, the medium tumor eyes were randomized (toss of a coin) to radiation treatment or prompt removal of the eye. The important result was to look at the rate the tumor going outside the eye and patient survival.

 At a ten and twenty year follow up, the COMS study showed that there was no difference in patient survival if the eye was treated with plaque radiation and preserved or if the eye was removed right away at the time of diagnosis.

WHAT HAPPENS IF I HAVE MELANOMA IN THE LIVER OR LUNGS?

As mentioned earlier, melanomas tend to stay confined to the eye for quite some time. Animal models have shown that the body develops immunity to the tumor cells (natural killer cells) that, theoretically at least, kill the tumor cells that are circulating in the blood stream.

However, at the time of initial diagnosis, it is imperative that a complete check up is done to look at the lungs, liver and other blood tests. If the tumor is present elsewhere, then the whole body needs to be treated. Specialty cancer centers and oncologists then prescribe treatment either chemotherapy, surgery or radiation. If during the follow up years, the tumor is discovered in the distant organs, once again the oncologists drive the treatment. There are several new melanoma drugs and trials that are available to patients at specialty cancer centers. Unfortunately, discovery of melanoma in the liver, lungs or elsewhere in the body reduces the life expectancy.

WHEN IS IT NOT A TUMOR?

There are a few conditions in the eye namely bleeding or blood clots or benign tumors that do not cause aggressive growth or loss of vision. Any time a mass is detected inside the eye, it needs to be examined by a specialist who can determine the characteristic signs a melanoma.

The most frequent conditions that mimic a melanoma are blood clots or a freckle in the eye (nevus) that can remain stable for a long period of time. In rare occasions, people who have cancers of the breast, lung or prostate can have disease that spreads to other parts of the body and, thus, can show up in small areas inside the eye.

Specialty ophthalmologists who deal with eye cancers can generally make the diagnosis by conducting the examinations listed in this handbook.

WHAT ABOUT A BENIGN TUMOR / CHOROIDAL NEVUS?

A large segment of the population, especially Caucasians, can have freckles in the eye. These are generally flat, pigmented areas in different parts of the back of the eye that can remain stable for a long period of time. Mostly, these are detected in a routine dilated eye exam, which prompts a referral to the specialist eye MD.

By conducting the tests listed above, mostly photographs and ultrasounds, these freckles can be monitored.

Sometimes a nevus of the choroid may appear suspicious for a small melanoma but doesn't fall into a clear-cut diagnosis. We look for the presence of 'tell-tale signs', namely whether there is leakage of fluid from the lesion, or there is an orange color or if it shows a growth along it's borders. In such situations, the doctor may examine you at three month intervals to be certain that early treatment can be started.

Generally, it is recommended that the follow-up dilated eye exams be conducted at least once a year. This is to ensure that if there is any slow growth, it can be treated with appropriate therapy at the right time.

CAN LASER BE USED TO TREAT MELANOMAS?

Laser can be used to treat small melanomas, but is generally kept as a supplemental treatment following radiation therapy. Laser treatment does have some side effects because it can leave blind spots in the eye and therefore is used judiciously.

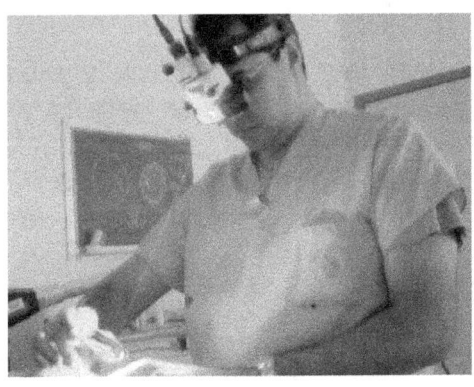

TREATMENT OF IRIS AND CILIARY BODY MELANOMAS

Iris melanomas are generally less aggressive in their growth. Quite often, they can remain stable for years at a time and can simply be observed during this time. If there is growth, they can cause glaucoma and cataract. Oftentimes, surgery to remove small tumors of the iris can cure or treat the tumor completely. The likelihood of iris tumors going outside the eye is very low.

Ciliary body tumors that remain hidden behind the lens of the eye are treated similarly to the choroid tumors, namely with radiation.

GENE EXPRESSION & GENETIC TYPING OF MELANOMAS

Over the last few years, specialty tests have been developed which provide genetic testing of the tumor cells. Generally, a small sample of the tumor is taken at the time of the radiation treatment by inserting a tiny needle through the sclera and sent to a specialty laboratory. Even a 0.1ml sample of tumor cells can provide enough material to run the gene expression analysis.

The most popular test available currently classifies the tumor cells into Type 1 (a or b) or Type 2. (Castle Bio Sciences). Another test looks at deletion of chromosome 3 (Univ. of Pennsylvania)

 Many studies have shown that Type 1 and Type 2 tumors have different characteristics of how they leave the eye. This reflects on the survival rate of the patient. Type 1 tumors tend to have a better prognosis in that the survival rate of the patient is close to 90% at a 5-year follow-up. On the other hand, survival rate of patients with Type 2 tumors is about 60% at a 5 year follow-up since these tumors tend to be more aggressive in leaving the eye and going to distance sites.

More and more genetic tests are being developed that will be able to further characterize the behavior of different types of melanomas that will be able to guide treatments, both for the eye and for the whole body.

SHOULD I EVEN DO GENETIC TYPING?
WHAT IF I DON'T WANT TO KNOW?
IS IT SAFE TO DO A BIOPSY?

Getting genetic typing done is a personal choice on the part of the patient. Many decide not to know what kind of tumor they have, whereas some patients want to know what their chances of 5-year survival are.

In a controlled, sterile environment like the operating room, it is safe to do the fine needle tumor biopsy.

Our practice is to encourage the patient to have the biopsy but leave it to their personal decision. Often this particular testing is not covered by insurance and can be expensive.

At this stage of our knowledge, the two strongest predictors of the tumor leading to distant metastases and thus survival over five years are: the tumor thickness (size) and whether it is type 1 or 2.

ENUCLEATION OF THE EYE

The first priority is to save the patient's life and avoid any unnecessary risks. The second priority is to save the eye as much as possible, and the third priority is to salvage as much vision as possible.

I like to advise patients that its similar to amputating a dead limb that has lost all use and may threaten their whole body. Painful and devastating but life saving.

Removal of the eye that has pain or complete loss of vision is sometimes necessary. If your doctor determines that the tumor is too far advanced or too big to be treated with radiation, the best treatment approach would then be removal of the eye. The reason for this is that if functional vision in that particular eye is already lost, and that the tumor is so big that there is a higher likelihood of it leaving the eye and going outside to distant organs, the best approach is to remove the eye that may potentially cause a danger to continued life expectancy.

While a decision is the hardest part as to whether the eye should be removed, the actual surgery is straightforward and can be life-saving. The surgery is done in the hospital since some patients will need an overnight stay. Mostly, the patient is put under general anesthesia. The eyelids are left intact and the eyeball is removed, preserving the muscles that rotate and move the eye. A ball implant is inserted where the eyeball was present and the muscles are stitched to the surface of the ball, which allows eye movement once the healing is complete. Since the volume of the orbit is replaced with the artificial ball, there is no shrinkage or abnormal appearance.

Following the surgery, expect there to be 2-3 weeks of swelling, pinkish discharge and scratchy discomfort until the healing process is completed. The pain can be moderate to severe in the first 24 hours, but after that most people do quite well with over-the-counter pain pills. We try to get a temporary artificial prosthesis (see below for more information) within the first 3-6 weeks following removal of the eye. This allows quick rehabilitation as well as a good cosmetic appearance.

One of the biggest challenges after removing the eye is the loss of peripheral vision in an eye that at least had some useful vision. It will take a major readjustment to become accustomed to using only one eye, however, the brain adapts very quickly so most people get back to near-normal activities. However, some patients may experience a 'ghost image' on that side, but this disappears after a few weeks.
We would strongly recommend reading the book called <u>A Singular View</u> by Frank Brady, who talks about getting used to depth perception and using one eye to perform most normal, everyday tasks.

PROSTHESIS FITTING

Getting a good match of a prosthesis for the eye that has been removed has come a long way over the last few years. Now, with newer technology, a very accurate color match can be made for the prosthesis. As mentioned above, once the swelling around the orbit has gone down, a specialty prosthesis maker will design a mold of the socket where the prosthesis will go.

(Photos courtesy of Jim Merritt, MD)

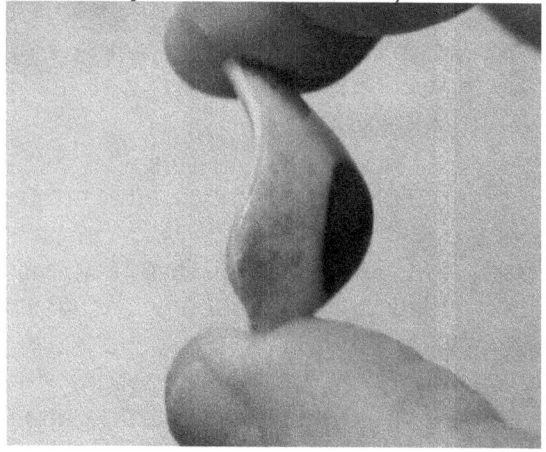

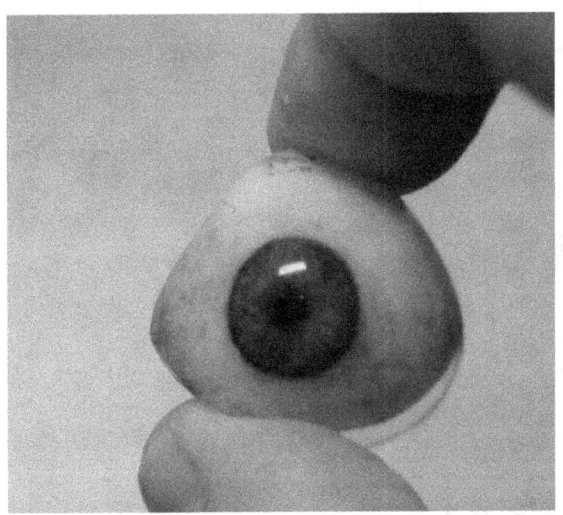

Generally, a temporary, colored contact lens can be placed within the eye to give a good cosmetic appearance while the rest of the healing is continuing. Prosthesis makers are artists who can color-match the exact pupil of the opposite side and even paint fine, red lines on the surface of the prosthesis that look like normal blood vessels. As long as there is some movement in the eyeball, most people cannot differentiate which eye is real and which eye is artificial.

Over the course of the years, the prosthesis will need to be adjusted and fine-tuned a little bit as a person grows and the eyelid becomes more lax. This is usually done within the first 1-2 years during follow-up and then the prosthesis maker can easily handle a good fitting.

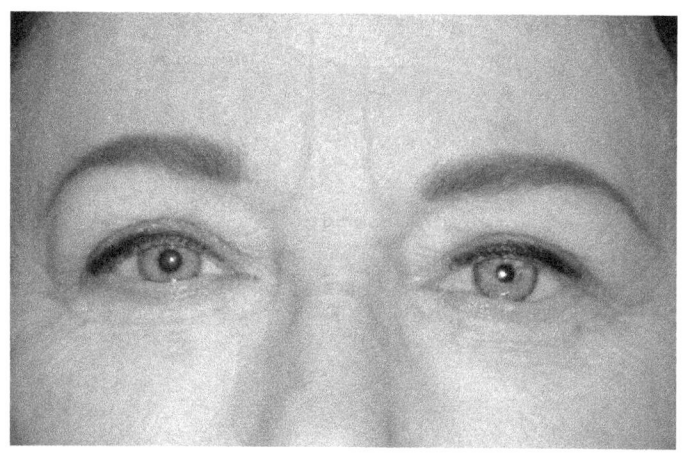

CONCLUSION

Melanomas of the eye are slow growing and therefore it is not an emergency to rush into action. As with any 'cancer' diagnosis, you will go through the stages of "shock, anger, resignation and acceptance". Then is the time to take a deep breath and realize that the condition is treatable.

After diagnosis, it is a good idea to carefully study the alternatives, risks and benefits of each treatment.

We hope that this short manual has given you some useful information as you make an informed decision as to how to proceed with treatment. As mentioned, once the treatment is initiated, most patients lead normal or near normal lives, even though they may lose some degree of vision.

The important factor is to continue the regular eye exams and medical follow up.

Continue reading the personal testimony of Dr. Jay Campbell, MD, who is a retina specialist and overcame his eye melanoma.

Good luck and God Bless!

PERSONAL TESTIMONY OF A RETINA DOCTOR

"When my eye melanoma was diagnosed I was 62 , in good health,
and a practicing ophthalmologist , in fact a retina specialist.

I was frightened and full of questions, not the least of which was why me , why does this eye doctor have a melanoma...the truthful answer is , why not me.
Why not accept the diagnosis
and look for the value in accepting
" what is" in my/ your life. And that is exactly what I did.

This excellent, informative handbook will answer many of your
questions. I wish one like this had been available to me .

My treatment prescribed by the doctors was plaque radiation therapy. The surgery and recovery
were much easier than I thought.
My full vision was saved and I returned to treating my patients

one week after the plaque was placed and the removed.
I was blessed with an excellent treatment team of physicians and
support staff.

I followed up with an oncologist,
and dilated eye exams per my doctor's orders.
Fortunately I practiced 5 more years after the melanoma was treated until
I retired in 2014. I've had no recurrence of the melanoma . I developed a cataract 4 years after melanoma treatment but that was easily surgically removed.

My initial fears of dying and losing my eye were very unwarranted and totally a waste of mind space.

As Dr Anand has so eloquently pointed out, at this time in medicine
ocular (eye) melanomas can be treated in a variety of effective ways
to preserve maximum sight and save the eye.

Now seven years later, I am melanoma free and a perfect 20/20
vision in both eyes.
I am indeed blessed and grateful to all of my

healers on this journey.

Oh yes , the value of having this melanoma happen to me I mentioned earlier.
The value was an increased empathy toward all my eye patients...indeed I was an eye patient too!!

Bless you on your path of treatment,
Jay Campbell MD

Acknowledgements

This book would not have come to be had it not been from the encouragement and comments I have received from my patients. It has been an honor to be able to help them through the course of their disease. Special thanks go to Lori C. for organizing the support group in Dallas-Fort Worth and the Melanoma Walk. I am indebted to my colleague and friend Jay Campbell for sharing his personal testimony.

We all stand on the shoulders of giants who have been pioneers in this field. I would especially like to thank my teachers Jerry Shields,MD and Jim Augsburger, MD who taught me so much during my stay at Wills Eye Hospital, Philadelphia. And of course, to Carol Shields, MD, who was my colleague and now has taken over the Oncology Service at Wills in her indomitable, hard-working fashion.

I have been indeed fortunate and blessed to have an expert group of retina colleagues at Texas Retina Associates in Dallas. In the field of melanoma management, who better than my associate Dr Dwain Fuller,MD,JD, as always for local expertise and wisdom.

My thanks to Cindy Funderbergh for help with the manuscript, and to my inimitable support staff Meredith Allen, Denise Reya, Ann Mungioli, and Jana Sierocki for their encouragement and assistance.

Resource list for patients

Collaborative Ocular Melanoma Study:
National Eye Institute
Melanoma Research Foundation
National Cancer Institute

Books from a patients perspective
A Singular view, Frank Brady
Eye was there, Slonim and Martino
Cure OM, Connie Robillard MA

Specialty Centers for Melanoma
(not a comprehensive list)
Wills Eye Hospital, Oncology Service,
Philadelphia, PA
Mayo Clinic, Rochester, MN
Cleveland Clinic, Cleveland, OH
UCLA, CA
Harvard Medical School, Boston, MA
Univ of San Francisco, CA

www.ingramcontent.com/pod-product-compliance
Lightning Source LLC
Chambersburg PA
CBHW070409190526
45169CB00003B/1176